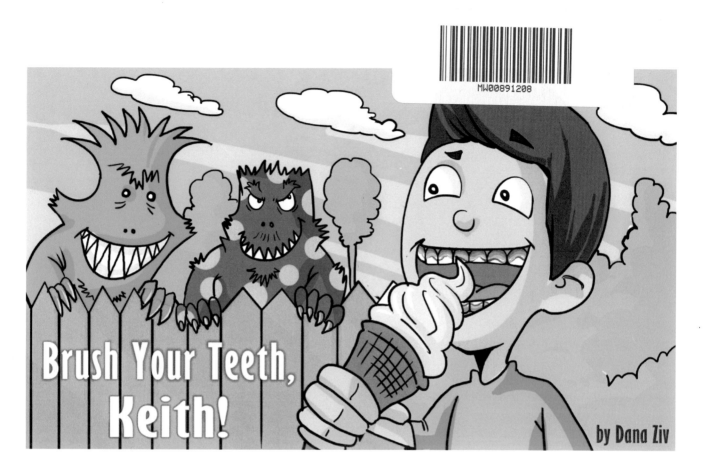

Brush Your Teeth, Keith!

Written by Dana Ziv

Illustrated by Abbas R.

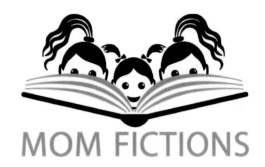

MOM FICTIONS

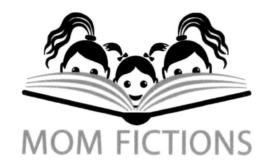

MOM FICTIONS

Thank you!
I had the privilege of writing this book with love, joy and real life passion.

I would love to read your thoughts and feelings about my book. your opinion matters!

With lots of love,
Dana

Please leave a review for "Brush Your Teeth, Keith!"

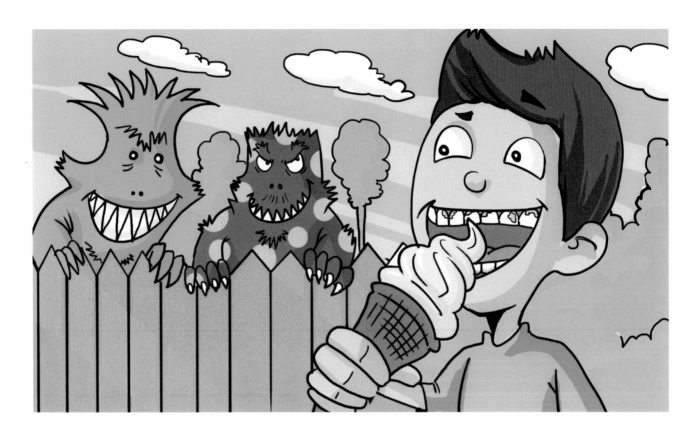

Brush Your Teeth, Keith!

Written by Dana Ziv
Illustrated by Abbas R.

Every morning and every night,
Keith refused to brush his teeth.
Mom would ask, but Keith would say,
 "No!" and stomp his feet.

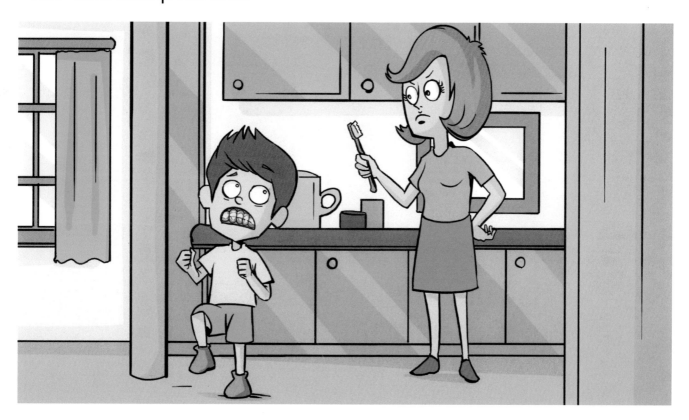

In the morning after the first meal,
Mommy urges him to brush, but still,
Keith refuses as he is certain,
brushing teeth is just a burden.

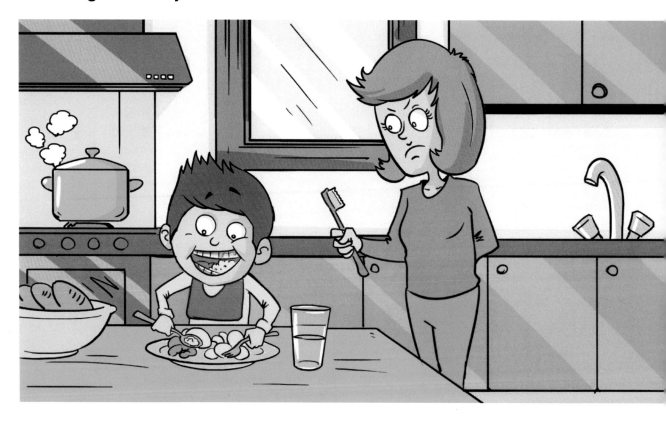

After dinner,
daddy is pulling the bed sheets for Keith.
Keith calmly climbs underneath,
Daddy asks him: "Did you brush your teeth?"

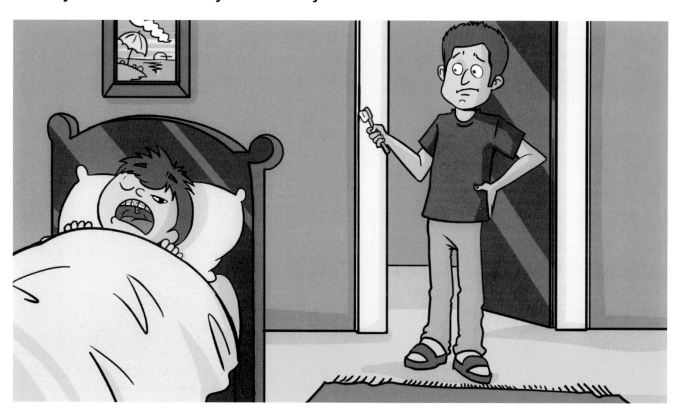

Keith looks a bit apprehensive,
and daddy feels a bit offensive.
"Good night" daddy says.
Places the toothbrush in the bathroom,
turns off the lights and walks to his bedroom.

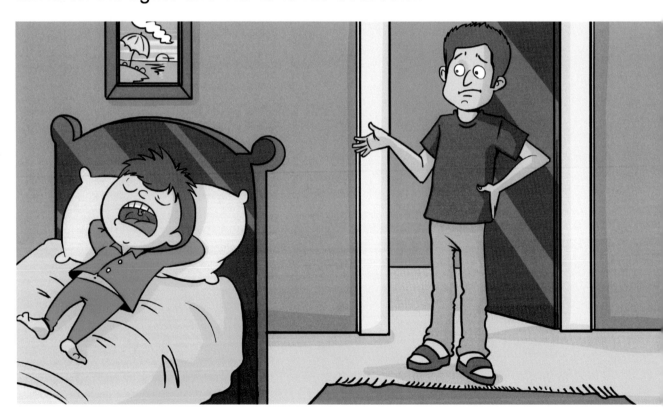

During the night, while Keith is fast asleep,
he hears voices coming from his teeth.
"Oh, this taste so good!", Someone sounds in a great mood.
And the other voice answers, "Best meal ever!"
"I hope Keith never brushes his teeth, so we can live here forever".
"This mouth is so dirty, and smells so bad, I simply love that!"

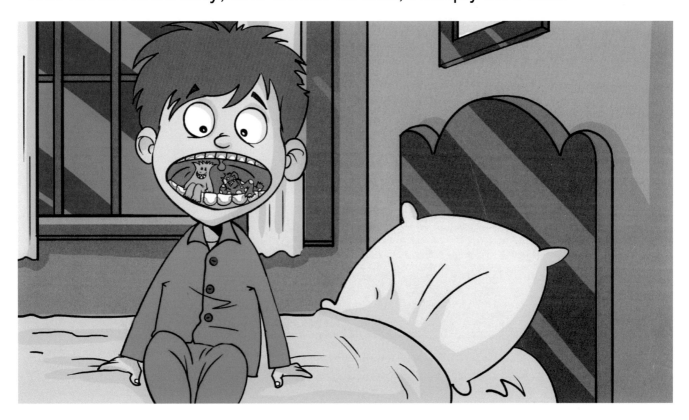

Keith quickly stands on his feet,
rushes to the mirror and looks at his teeth.
staring closely in the mirror,
he sees two creatures playing together.
He starts to shiver.
Keith cannot believe his eyes,
and screams out loud, "Who are you guys?!"

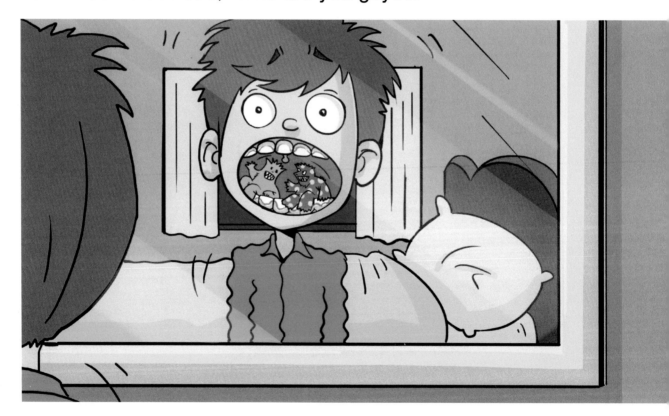

Mickey and Mooch look at each other,
swallow hard and say, "Um…we are brothers".
"We came to look for a new home, the dirtiest and smelliest we
could roam."
"And everybody in town has been saying Keith's mouth is the best,"
they are explaining.

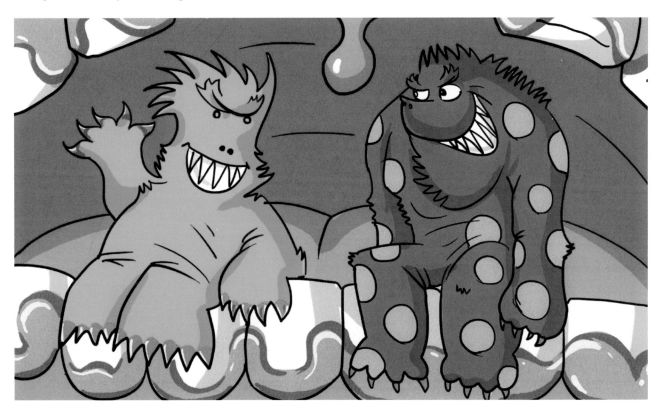

Keith is shocked.
He cannot believe his ears and eyes.
He rushes to the bathroom, closes the door,
pulls out his tooth paste,
and starts brushing more and more.
Mickey and Mooch go down the drain,
Keith does not want to see them ever again.

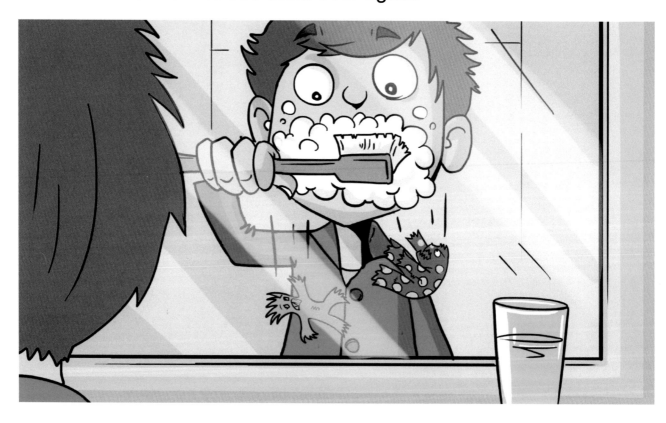

The next day it is no longer necessary.
Keith does not need a secretary.
The first thing he does after getting up,
is brush his teeth and rinse with a cup.
The same drill continues at night.
Mom and Dad cannot believe their sight.

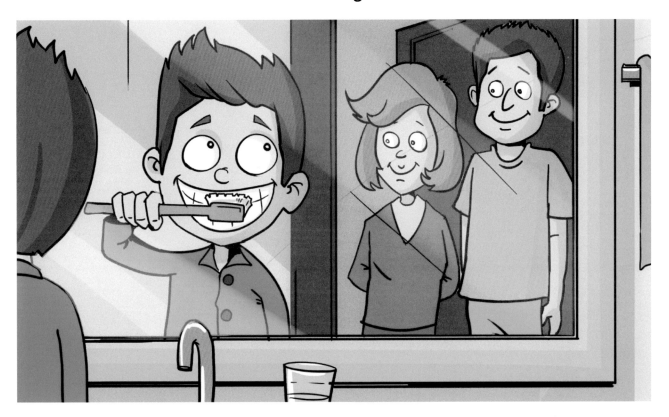

And it continues to this day,
Keith keeps his mouth clean and brushes twice a day.

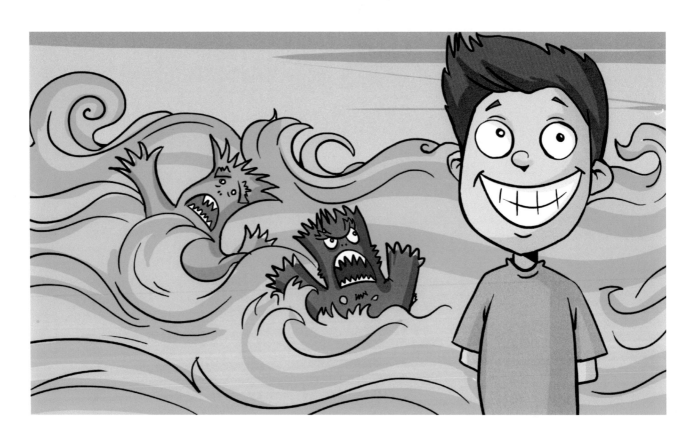

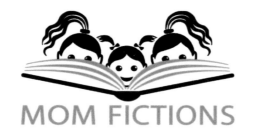

MOM FICTIONS

Thank you!
I had the privilege of writing this book with love, joy and real life passion.

I would love to read your thoughts and feelings about my book. your opinion matters!

With lots of love,
Dana

Please leave a review for "Brush Your Teeth, Keith!"

A complete Read Along Video version is waiting for you.

My gift to you!
go to : http://www.momfictions.com/#!promo/hcig6

Enjoy!

Please feel free to reach me directly
for any comments, questions or feedback:
momfictions@gmail.com

Or visit us at: www.momfictions.com

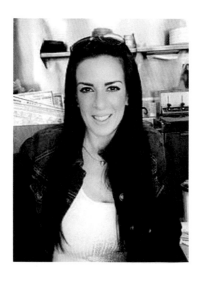

Your's Truly,
Dana Ziv

Overview

Take good care of your child's baby teeth. They do eventually fall out but until they do, baby teeth play an important role in helping your child bite and chew food, and speak clearly. Many of the same treatment and evaluation options that adults have are also available to kids. These include X-rays, dental sealants, orthodontic treatment and more.

What to Expect During Childhood

Wiggly teeth

When a child is about 6 years old, his/her teeth will begin to come loose. Let your child wiggle the tooth until it falls out on its own. This will minimize the pain and bleeding associate with a lost tooth.

Cavities

Cavities can develop when sugar-containing foods are allowed to stay in the mouth for a long time.

Bacteria that live on the teeth feast on these bits of food and can eat away at tooth enamel. Saliva washes away the acid between meals, but if your child is always eating, there may not be time for this acid to get washed away.

Parents: The Best Role Models

Parents play an important role in their children's dental health. They need to reinforce good oral hygiene habits such as brushing and flossing at home with their children.

However, the most important impact on your children will come from observing your own good habits. Lead by example and demonstrate how important your children's teeth are to their overall health and continuing quality of life. Optimal dental health translates to a healthier child in general and impacts their future habits and livelihood.

Brush your Teeth, Keith! Word MIX-UP

There are a lot of different ways to keep your mouth healthy.

Unscramble these words to reveal things that can help keep your smile sparkling.

1. OUTBTSORHH _____ Hint: Replace this every three months.

2. HSTTTAEOOP _____ Hint: Squeeze just a bit on toothbrush.

3. OLSFS _____ Hint: Use 18 inches of this once a day.

4. HYHTAEL DOOF _____ Hint: includes fruits, veggies & milk.

5. DSNTTIE _____ Hint: Visit him/her every six months.

6. REFODLIU _____ Hint: all you need is a quick swish.

7. HMOWHTUSA _____ Hint: This helps fight cavities, so make sure it's in your toothpaste and mouth rinse or ask your dentist for more information.

Answers: 1.Toothbrush 2.Toothpaste 3.Floss 4.Healthy Food 5.Dentist 6.Flouride 7.Mouthwash

Word Search

T	D	E	N	T	I	S	T
Y	E	X	A	M	B	H	O
T	N	E	R	L	F	S	O
I	T	F	T	A	I	U	T
V	A	L	N	H	Y	R	H
A	L	O	G	S	O	B	F
C	V	F	A	M	D	P	A
F	I	L	L	I	N	G	I
R	S	O	P	L	D	S	R
D	I	S	D	E	C	A	Y
M	T	S	A	K	L	I	M

dentist / exam / teeth / cavity / floss / dental visit / tooth fairy / filling / x-ray / smile / milk / decay / brush

Enjoy Coloring Keith while he is brushing his teeth

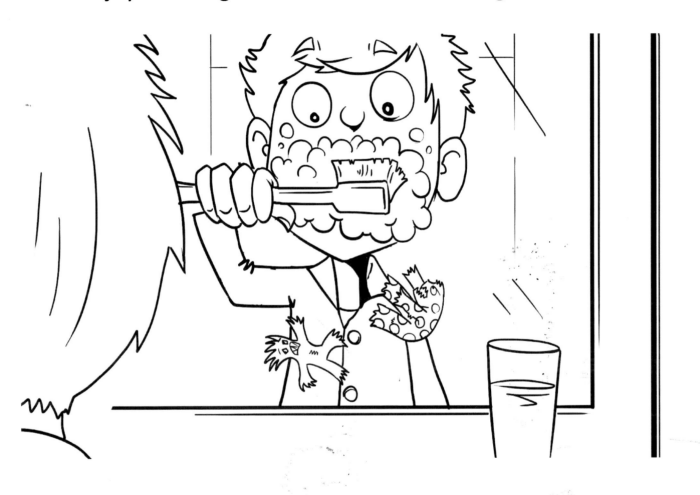

For the latest books by Dana Ziv

Go to www.momfictions.com

Coming Soon!

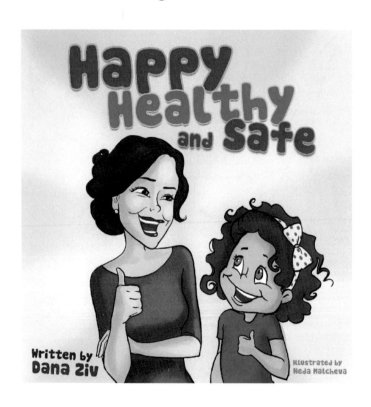

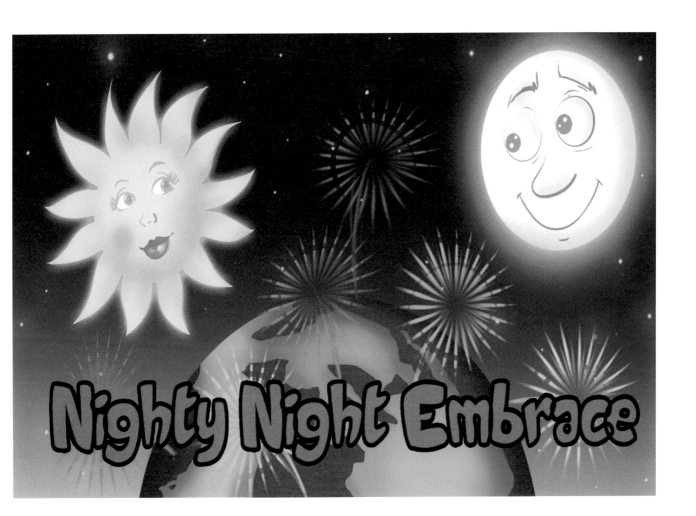

THE END

Made in the USA
Middletown, DE
18 April 2017